FIGHT AGAINST BREAST CANCER WITH BALANCED DIET MEAL PLAN

An Ultimate and Recommended 30-Days Diet Meal Plan Natural Remedies for Surviving and Prevention of Breast Cancer

ADAM FIDELIS

TABLE OF CONTENT

INTRODUCTION

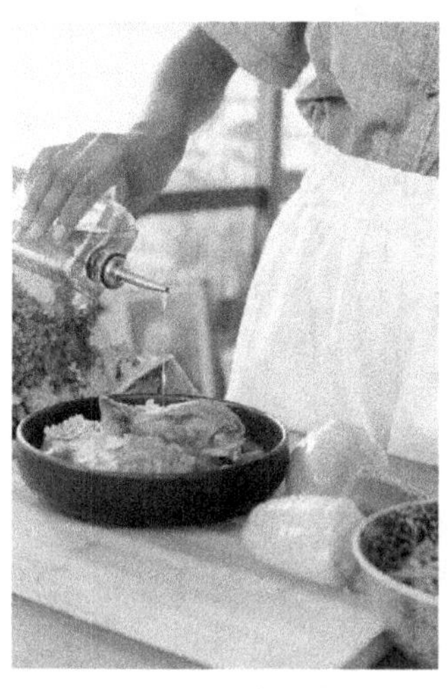

Julie found an unexpected ally in her fight against breast cancer in the small village of Serenity Springs: her kitchen. Determined to add a holistic element to her medical treatment, Julie adopted a well-planned diet meal plan. She assembled a nutrient-dense dish, topped with lush greens, lean proteins, and vibrant fruits, following the advice of nutritionists to bolster her immune system. Her anti-inflammatory armor was made of curries infused with turmeric. Berries, being high in antioxidants, provided Julie with comfort as they fought off free radicals, which posed a threat to her health.

Green tea's polyphenols were fighting cancer cells as she consumed it. Her story is a testament to the significance of a well-balanced diet in the fight against breast cancer, and it involved more than simply meals. Julie discovered that feeding her body was a powerful weapon when she was surrounded by the aroma of healthful foods, transforming her kitchen into a haven of resilience and optimism in the face of hardship.

BREAST CANCER DIET MEAL PLAN

Day 1: Meal and preparation

Breakfast: Berry Smoothie

Ingredients:

1 cup mixed berries (blueberries, strawberries, raspberries)

1/2 cup Greek yogurt

1 tablespoon flaxseeds

Preparation:

Blend mixed berries, Greek yogurt, and flaxseeds until smooth. Customize with a splash of almond milk for consistency.

Day 2: Meal and preparation

Lunch: Quinoa Salad

Ingredients:

1 cup quinoa

2 cups spinach

1 cup cherry tomatoes, halved

1/2 avocado, diced

Preparation:

Cook quinoa and let it cool. Toss with fresh spinach, cherry tomatoes, and avocado. Drizzle with olive oil and a squeeze of lemon for added flavor.

Day 3: Meal and preparation

Dinner: Grilled Salmon

Ingredients:

6 oz salmon fillet

1 lemon, sliced

2 cloves garlic, minced

1 teaspoon rosemary, chopped

Preparation:

Marinate salmon with minced garlic, rosemary, and lemon slices. Grill until the salmon is cooked to perfection.

Day 4: Meal and preparation

Snack: Greek Yogurt Parfait

Ingredients:

1 cup Greek yogurt

1/2 cup granola

1/2 cup mixed berries (blueberries, strawberries)

Preparation:

Layer Greek yogurt, granola, and mixed berries in a glass for a delightful parfait.

Day 5: Meal and preparation

Breakfast: Oatmeal with Walnuts

Ingredients:

1/2 cup oats

1 cup almond milk

2 tablespoons walnuts

1/2 teaspoon cinnamon

Preparation:

Cook oats in almond milk, top with chopped walnuts, and sprinkle cinnamon for added taste.

Day 6: Meal and preparation

Lunch: Spinach and Chickpea Salad

Ingredients:

1 can chickpeas, drained and rinsed

2 cups spinach

1 cup cherry tomatoes, halved

1/2 cup feta cheese, crumbled

Preparation:

Combine chickpeas, spinach, cherry tomatoes, and crumbled feta cheese. Drizzle with olive oil for a finishing touch.

Day 7: Meal and preparation

Dinner: Stir-Fried Broccoli and Tofu

Ingredients:

1 cup broccoli florets

1/2 block tofu, cubed

2 tablespoons soy sauce

1 teaspoon ginger, minced

Preparation:

Stir-fry tofu and broccoli in soy sauce and minced ginger until cooked to your liking.

Day 8: Meal and preparation

Snack: Almond and Cranberry Trail Mix

Ingredients:

1/2 cup almonds

1/4 cup dried cranberries

2 tablespoons pumpkin seeds

Preparation:

Mix almonds, dried cranberries, and pumpkin seeds. Portion into snack-sized bags for a convenient, on-the-go treat.

Day 9: Meal and preparation

Breakfast: Chia Seed Pudding

Ingredients:

2 tablespoons chia seeds

1 cup almond milk

Kiwi slices

Preparation:

Mix chia seeds with almond milk and refrigerate overnight. Top with kiwi slices before serving.

Day 10: Meal and preparation

Lunch: Lentil Soup

Ingredients:

1 cup lentils

1 cup carrots, diced

1/2 cup celery, chopped

1/2 cup onion, diced

Preparation:

Cook lentils with diced carrots, celery, and onions in a flavorful broth.

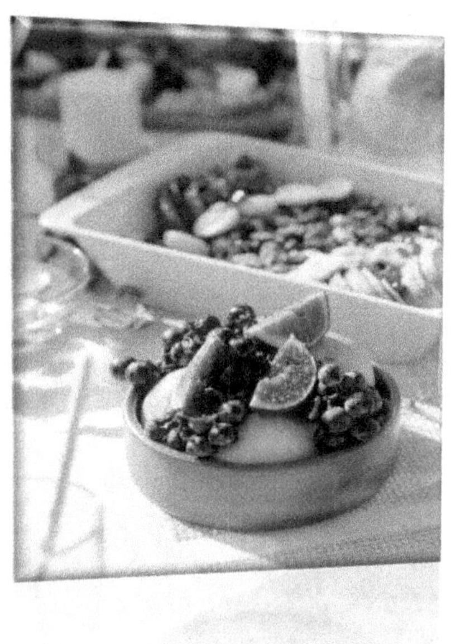

Day 11: Meal and preparation

Dinner: Baked Chicken with Sweet Potatoes

Ingredients:

6 oz chicken breast

1 sweet potato, sliced

1 tablespoon olive oil

1 teaspoon rosemary

Preparation:

Season chicken and sweet potatoes with olive oil and rosemary, then bake until fully cooked.

Day 12: Meal and preparation

Snack: Carrot Sticks with Hummus

Ingredients:

Carrot sticks

Hummus

Preparation:

Simply dip carrot sticks into hummus for a satisfying and nutritious snack.

Day 13: Meal and preparation

Breakfast: Avocado Toast with Poached Egg

Ingredients:

2 slices whole-grain bread

1/2 avocado

1 poached egg

Preparation:

Spread mashed avocado on toasted bread and top with a perfectly poached egg.

Day 14: Meal and preparation

Lunch: Brown Rice Bowl with Vegetables

Ingredients:

1 cup brown rice

1 cup broccoli

1/2 cup bell peppers, sliced

2 tablespoons soy sauce

Preparation:

Stir-fry veggies and toss with cooked brown rice. Drizzle with soy sauce for a tasty bowl.

Day 15: Meal and preparation

Dinner: Grilled Shrimp Skewers

Ingredients:

8 oz shrimp

1 lemon, squeezed

2 cloves garlic, minced

1 tablespoon olive oil

Preparation:

Marinate shrimp with lemon, minced garlic, and olive oil, then grill on skewers until cooked.

Continue to adjust portions based on individual needs, and consult with healthcare professionals or nutritionists for personalized advice and adjustments.

Day 16: Meal and preparation

Snack: Apple Slices with Almond Butter

Ingredients:

1 medium apple, sliced

2 tablespoons almond butter

Preparation:

Spread almond butter on apple slices for a satisfying and nutritious snack.

Day 17: Meal and preparation

Breakfast: Greek Yogurt Pancakes

Ingredients:

1 cup whole-grain flour

1/2 cup Greek yogurt

1 egg

Preparation:

Mix whole-grain flour, Greek yogurt, and egg. Cook pancakes and serve with a dollop of yogurt.

Day 18: Meal and preparation

Lunch: Quinoa and Black Bean Bowl

Ingredients:

1 cup quinoa

1 can black beans, drained and rinsed

1/2 cup corn

1 lime

Preparation:

Cook quinoa, mix with black beans and corn. Squeeze lime for a refreshing taste.

Day 19: Meal and preparation

Dinner: Baked Cod with Asparagus

Ingredients:

6 oz cod fillet

1 bunch asparagus

1 lemon

1 teaspoon dill

Preparation:

Season cod and asparagus with lemon and dill, then bake until fully cooked.

Day 20: Meal and preparation

Snack: Cottage Cheese with Pineapple

Ingredients:

1/2 cup cottage cheese

1/2 cup fresh pineapple, diced

Preparation:

Mix cottage cheese with pineapple chunks for a balanced and tasty snack.

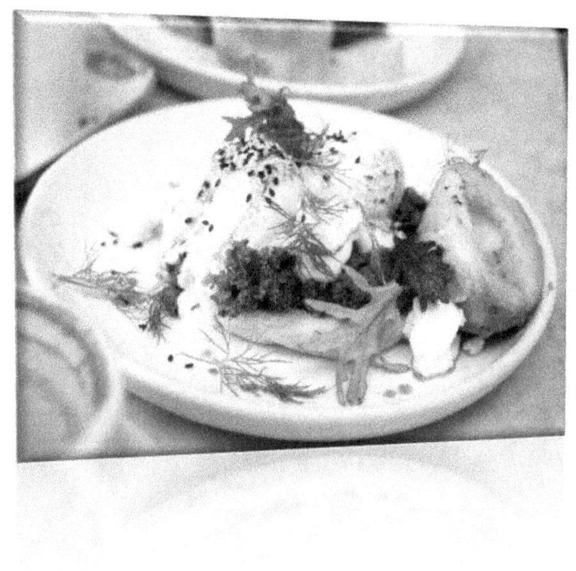

Day 21: Meal and preparation

Breakfast: Spinach and Feta Omelet

Ingredients:

3 eggs

1 cup spinach, chopped

1/4 cup feta cheese, crumbled

Preparation:

Whisk eggs, add spinach and feta, then cook into a delicious omelet.

Day 22: Meal and preparation

Lunch: Turkey and Avocado Wrap

Ingredients:

1 whole-grain wrap

3 oz turkey slices

1/2 avocado, sliced

Handful of lettuce

Preparation:

Layer turkey, avocado, and lettuce, then wrap it up for a quick and nutritious lunch.

Day 23: Meal and preparation

Dinner: Eggplant and Chickpea Curry

Ingredients:

1 medium eggplant, diced

1 can chickpeas, drained and rinsed

2 tomatoes, diced

Curry spices (turmeric, cumin, coriander)

Preparation:

Cook eggplant, chickpeas, and tomatoes with a blend of curry spices for a hearty curry.

Day 24: Meal and preparation

Snack: Blueberry and Almond Smoothie

Ingredients:

1 cup blueberries

1 cup almond milk

2 tablespoons almond butter

Preparation:

Blend blueberries, almond milk, and almond butter for a creamy and nutritious smoothie.

Day 25: Meal and preparation

Breakfast: Overnight Chia Seed Pudding with Mango

Ingredients:

3 tablespoons chia seeds

1 cup almond milk

1 mango, diced

Preparation:

Mix chia seeds with almond milk and refrigerate overnight. Top with diced mango before serving.

Day 26: Meal and preparation

Lunch: Tomato Basil Mozzarella Salad

Ingredients:

2 tomatoes, sliced

4 oz fresh mozzarella, sliced

Fresh basil leaves

Balsamic vinaigrette

Preparation:

Layer tomato and mozzarella slices with fresh basil leaves. Drizzle with balsamic vinaigrette for a refreshing salad.

Day 27: Meal and preparation

Dinner: Stir-Fried Tofu with Broccoli and Brown Rice

Ingredients:

1/2 block tofu, cubed

1 cup broccoli florets

1 cup brown rice, cooked

2 tablespoons soy sauce

Preparation:

Stir-fry tofu and broccoli, then toss with cooked brown rice and soy sauce for a tasty and balanced meal.

Day 28: Meal and preparation

Snack: Kale Chips

Ingredients:

1 bunch kale, stems removed

1 tablespoon olive oil

Sea salt to taste

Preparation:

Toss kale in olive oil, sprinkle with sea salt, and bake until crispy for a nutritious and crunchy snack.

Day 29: Meal and preparation

Breakfast: Whole-Grain Waffles with Strawberries

Ingredients:

2 whole-grain waffles

1 cup fresh strawberries, sliced

Preparation:

Toast whole-grain waffles and top with sliced strawberries for a delicious and wholesome breakfast.

Day 30: Meal and preparation

Lunch: Salmon Salad with Avocado

Ingredients:

6 oz grilled salmon

2 cups mixed greens

1/2 avocado, sliced

Lemon for dressing

Preparation:

Flake grilled salmon over a bed of mixed greens, top with avocado slices, and squeeze lemon for a refreshing dressing.

CONCLUSION

In conclusion, our group's experience using a well-chosen diet to combat breast cancer is proof of the revolutionary power of mindful eating. It represents more than just a diet; it's our dedication to bolstering our resilience in the face of hardship and advancing general health.

Every nutrient-dense item contains a potent defense against the obstacles posed by cancer in addition to nourishment. Our bodies are strengthened and our immune systems are boosted by the antioxidants, proteins, and variety of vitamins included in the foods we have chosen.

This is a commitment to enhancing our resilience and well-being, not just a diet plan. With every thoughtful decision we make, we reaffirm our commitment to living a robust and vibrant life. It's an honoring of the resilience of the human spirit and a recognition that each mouthful of food is a step toward a better life.

By adopting this diet plan, we affirm that the battle against breast cancer involves not just medical treatments but also our everyday decisions. By feeding with meaning and purpose, we light the way to recovery and resilience.

As we move forward, let our determination remain unshaken. Inspired by the potential for transformation embedded in our dietary choices, we stride confidently toward a future where wellness triumphs over adversity. Together, we exemplify the potency of nutrition in the relentless pursuit of health and life, standing united against breast cancer's challenges.

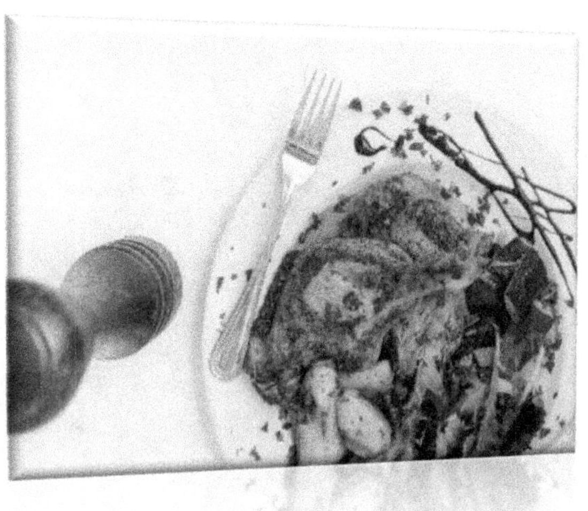

Stay healthy!!!